Red Light Therapy

Daniel Jackson

Red Light Therapy

© Daniel Jackson 2022 All Rights Reserved

The moral right of the author has been asserted

First published by Rockwood Publishing 2022

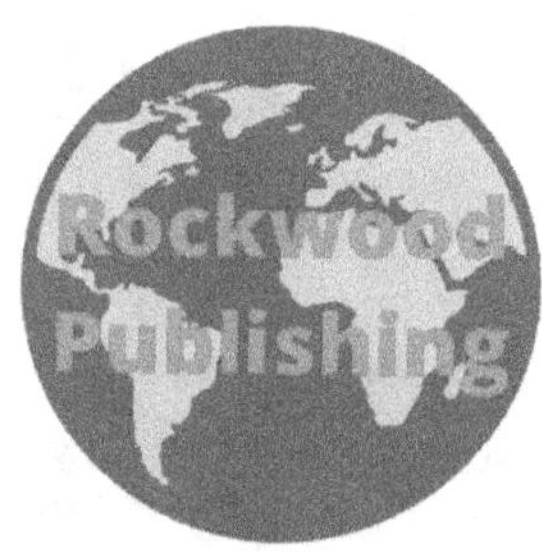

Contents

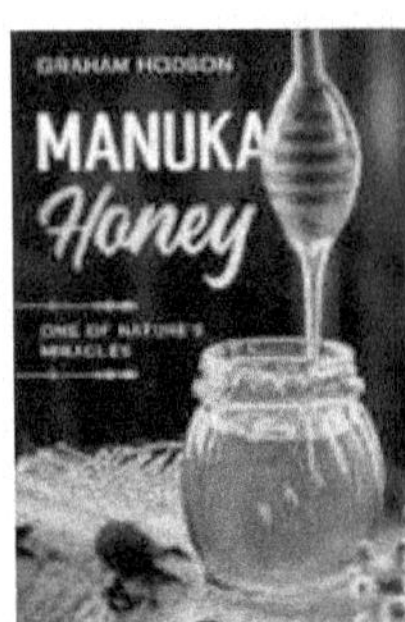
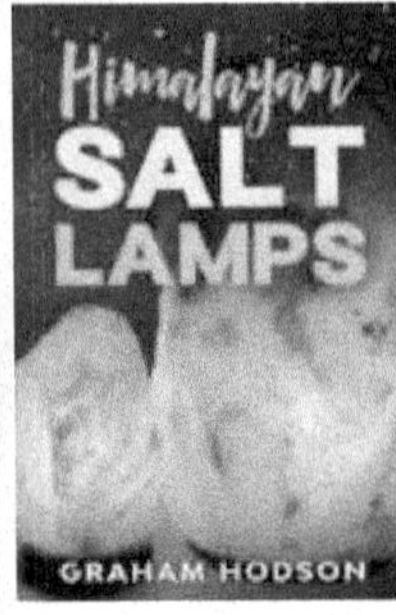
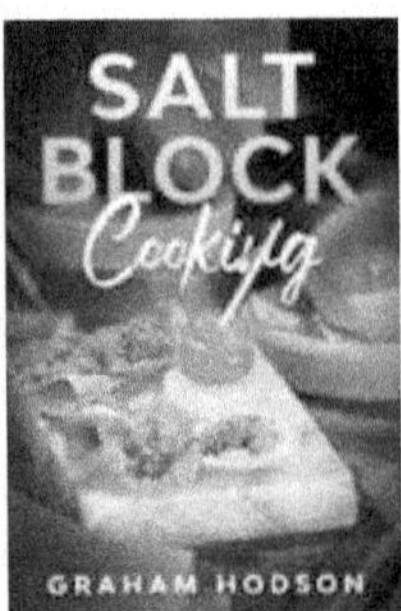
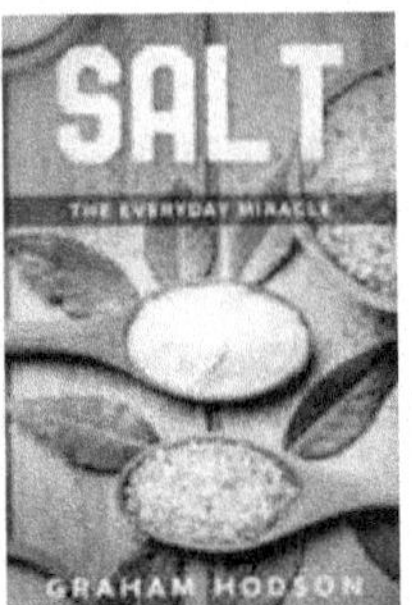

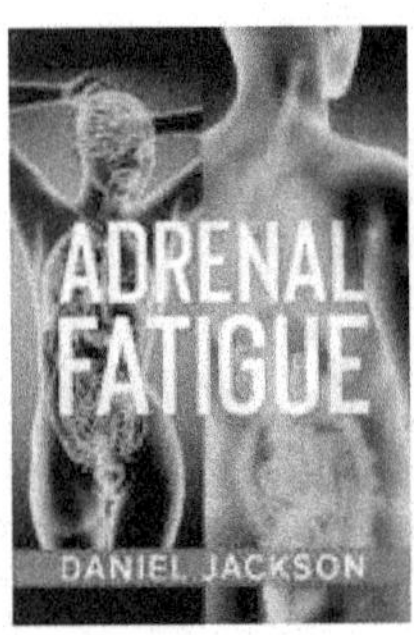
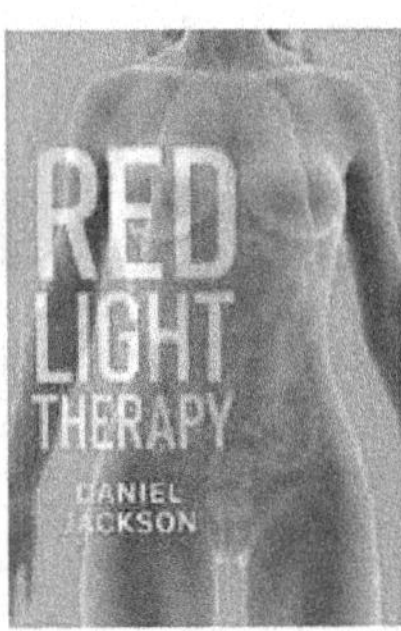
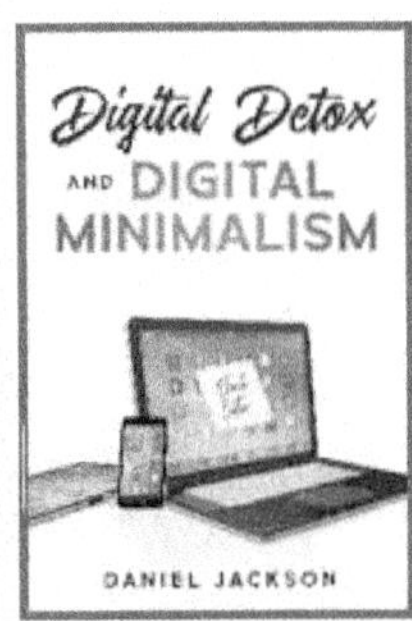
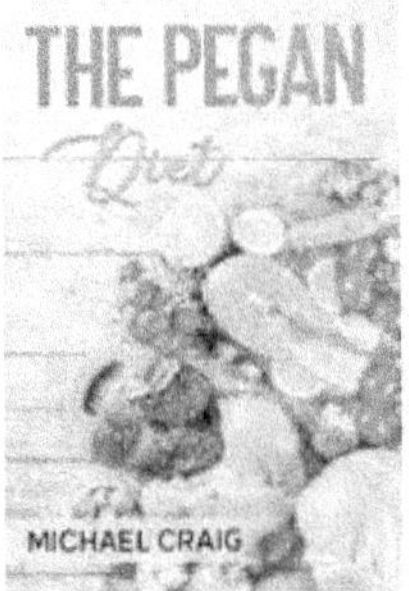

Take a look at more great books available from Rockwood Publishing

… some for FREE!

Just visit the link below:

rockwoodpublishing.co.uk

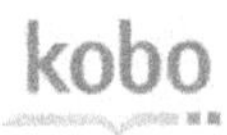
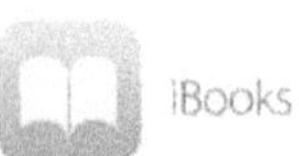

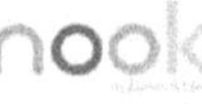
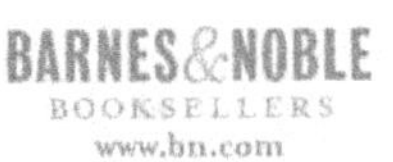

Introduction

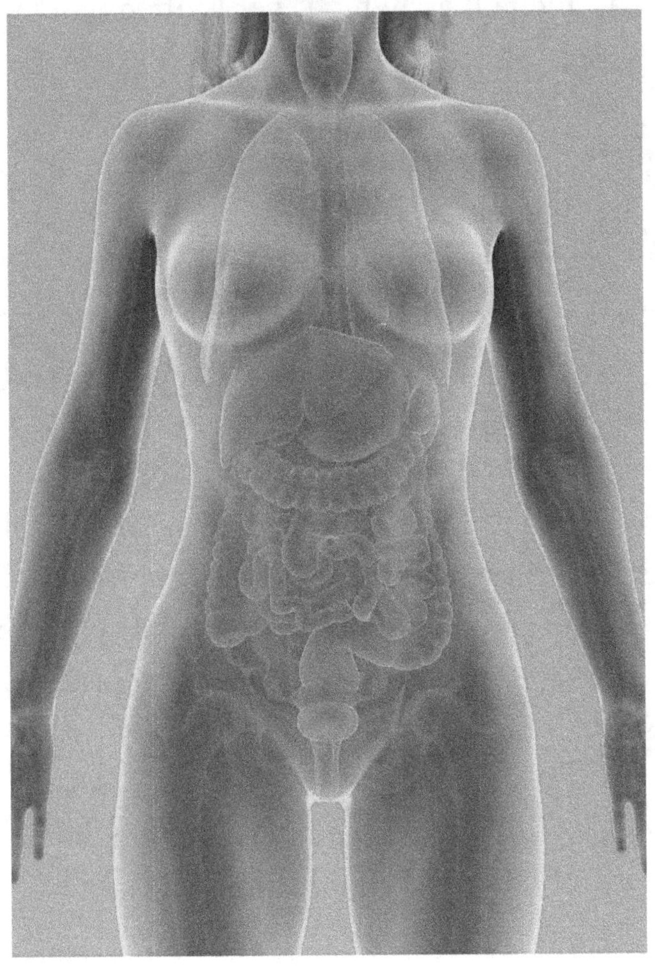

With each passing year, our understanding of the ways that we can promote wellness and prevent disease via natural methods grows, and this is why red light therapy has become such a catalyst for health-conscious individuals looking to improve their quality of life without having to rely on pharmaceutical drugs or other traditional medicines which very often come with countless side effects.

Red light therapy is a natural, economical, and effective way to heal and repair your body.

It's also an alternative solution that you can easily use in conjunction with other treatments so you can potentially enjoy faster recovery times.

I *don't* see it as the be-all, end-all, cure-all miracle treatment (because nothing is!), but rather as one of many beneficial natural therapies that can help improve health and wellness when used appropriately and responsibly.

This book is for you if you are looking for a safe, natural way to improve your health.

Daniel Jackson

What is Red Light Therapy?

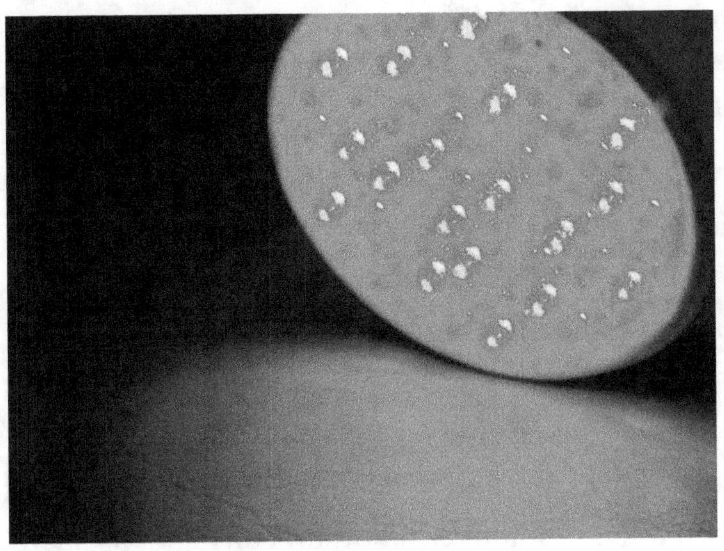

Light therapy's health advantages are nothing new. People used it in the late 1800s to treat tuberculosis, and NASA utilized it in the 1980s to cultivate plants in space. It has also been a part of professional or at-home skincare treatments for quite some time.

Light therapy works by visible light penetrating through the skin that is then absorbed by the cells in your body.

Different colors of light have different wavelengths, which means some are better at treating certain conditions more effectively than others. Red light is one of the best colors when it comes to treating common health problems.

Red light therapy, sometimes referred to as red laser therapy or infrared heat treatment, uses a particular natural wavelength of light for therapeutic purposes, both medical and cosmetic. It is derived from an infrared light source that also emits heat.

There is a wide range of visible light frequencies and wavelengths of light. Red light at its wavelength is known to be bio-active in human cells and, as such, can directly and specifically influence and enhance cellular function.

Our skin is permeable to red light, which means it can get into the deeper layers called the dermis. When light enters the cells, it is absorbed and transformed into cellular energy.

It's actually the photons in red light that are able to penetrate deep into the tissue, and this process works on a molecular level to stimulate ATP production (the aforementioned cellular energy).

It can also increase circulation and collagen synthesis, which has positive benefits for the skin.

Red light also suppresses inflammation by decreasing leukotrienes and prostaglandin PGE2 production, and can also increase cellular oxygen, which helps to detoxify cells. So, in other words, by increasing the oxygenation process, red light further enhances metabolic function and tissue repair.

It also has an antibacterial effect by stimulating white blood cells responsible for fighting infection within the body.

Red light energy also increases nitric oxide production and therefore has what's referred to as a vasodilating effect.

This helps with skin conditions such as psoriasis because it allows the capillaries to open up and increase blood flow within the skin, while at the same time reducing redness and inflammation.

Types of Red Light Therapy

Today, alternative kinds of red light therapy (RLT) are available and these different therapy types positively affect conditions like acne, hyperhidrosis, psoriasis, and many other skin disorders.

One can use red light therapy in the form of lasers and LED lights to treat specific medical conditions.

A brief explanation of each type will help you understand how this modality works as it's important that you know what kind of therapy is best to adopt, and not just go for any form of red light therapy.

Photobiomodulation (PBM)

This is the most common type of red light therapy and is used for various disorders. PBM has been used to treat psoriasis, acne, diabetic ulcers, and many neurodegenerative diseases, and the treatment uses LED light to generate both red and near-infrared light.

The wavelengths of the two are different, but they both have beneficial effects on cell activity.

It's important not to confuse PBM with low-level laser therapy (LLLT).

The mechanism of action of PBM has been studied in detail by researchers and scientists all over the world and the therapy works in two ways: -

i)   it increases cell energy production
ii)   it increases blood flow to the affected area

Both of these actions help reduce pain and promote tissue regeneration.

Therapies that use PBM are known to increase ATP levels in the cells which is the molecule involved in cellular metabolism.

Low-level laser therapy (LLLT)

This is another form of red light therapy that uses lasers to treat psoriasis, acne, wounds, and carpal tunnel syndrome, but the treatment is mainly used for musculoskeletal problems. However, it is effective in treating almost all conditions that respond positively to photobiomodulation.

LLLT also emits red light wavelengths that are beneficial to cell activity, but the light has a lower intensity than that of PBM.

Cold Laser Therapy

The majority of superficial tissue is treated with wavelengths between 600nm and 700nm. Wider penetration is obtained utilizing wavelengths ranging from 780nm to 950nm.
This is known as cold laser therapy.

During cold laser therapy, a low power level is used to treat injuries and various musculoskeletal conditions.

The treatment can be administered in several ways: -

i) the concentrated beam of light may be applied on top of or underneath the skin directly onto the affected area. This mode will provide *direct* results.

ii) The light may be applied to the skin overlying specific acupuncture points. This mode will *indirectly* promote healing and pain relief.

iii)   A laser probe can be inserted transcutaneously into the affected area using a hypodermic needle. This mode gives a more focused treatment since it does not have to travel through the layers of tissue before reaching its target.

In general, the treatment does not cause pain but increases local circulation significantly and, as such, delivers cellular energy much faster. In other words, it speeds up the rate at which cells heal by stimulating metabolic processes and blood flow in the affected area.

A person should always opt for cold laser therapy if there are any doubts about the safety of PBM therapy or the LLLT.

These two treatments are generally known to be safe, but the former can occasionally have side effects in some instances.

Red Light Therapy Precautions and Tips

Patients who opt for red light therapy should follow specific tips and techniques in order to gain the greatest benefit.

Before they begin their course of treatment, they should make themselves familiar with any precautions and safety measures that doctors or therapists use. This helps to avoid any potential setbacks during treatments.

It is vital to follow all safety measures, and to not miss any appointments so as to prevent any setbacks in recovery.

Also, patients need to be fully aware of the status of their own health.

Self-care is essential for recovering from any chronic health condition. The ideal location in which the therapy takes place is a dark room with comfortable chairs and/or a couch that can be used should you need to lie down on during treatment.

The area should be well ventilated to avoid any heat build-up in the room in order to minimize the possibility of dehydration.

As already stated, it is essential that you consult with your health care provider/doctor ***before*** you start any treatment.

The therapy should only ever be administered under a doctor's supervision or by an approved/certified therapist.

The safest way to receive red light therapy is by going through an approved center since this ensures the quality of equipment used and procedures performed.

Patients should also be on the lookout for "red flags" when it comes to finding a treatment center. They should ask questions and avoid centers that are not transparent about the process, or that use equipment that is not certified.

The person undergoing therapy needs to wear loose, comfortable clothing during treatment, and without any metal buttons or zips.

The patient/practitioner should cover the area being treated with a towel and possibly use oil-free lotion as a way to help them relax.

Always remember that the treatment should be stopped if they develop any symptoms that are unusual.

It's vital to drink lots of water during healing sessions, as this helps with flushing out toxins from the body and boosts blood circulation. Patients are usually advised to consume at least six glasses of water in order to aid their recovery.

They should also be encouraged to eat healthy meals and generally take in food that is rich in essential nutrients.

Patients are advised not to apply sunscreen on the area that has been treated with red light therapy. The skin should also be protected from the sun's rays and extreme temperatures for about 48 hours after treatment so that it can heal properly.

This is because red light therapy by its very nature is known to cause vasodilation and increase blood flow to the affected area which makes the skin more sensitive to sunlight and other forms of heat that may in turn cause injuries to, or scars on, the skin.

Before beginning red light therapy, choosing a suitable location that provides privacy during treatment is essential. This could be at home, but in this case it's important that all members of the household agree to follow all safety measures.

Many people choose to attend alternative therapy centers that are specifically designed for such therapies. A person undergoing red light therapy should not drink alcohol, smoke, or take any medication or recreational drugs before the treatment session.

They mustn't consume caffeine as this interferes with the metabolism of cells and slows down cellular energy production.

Patients are advised to avoid any stressful situations that may hamper their recovery.

Before treatment commences, the ideal emotional state is one of feeling relaxed and calm.

Also, it is essential to have patience when trying out red light therapy as the results are not usually immediate and indeed may take some time.

There may also be visible changes in skin tone after a few sessions of therapy.

How is a Therapy Session Conducted?

There is no set method by which a therapy session must be conducted, as the patient's wishes and needs are paramount, individual, and, as such, put first. However, to expose the skin to red light for a long enough period to work on an area or condition, you may want to follow these steps:

a) You will most likely have a consultation with your therapist before you begin in order to discuss the areas that need most work and which sites are suitable for red light therapy. You may be required to fill in a form with details of any medications you're taking or other medical conditions you have.

b) You will likely be supplied with a gown-type garment, as it is essential that the area you are treating is exposed in order for the light to be absorbed into your skin.

The treatment room will have been set up and the equipment tested long before you arrive, so it's generally a case of removing any clothing from the area to receive treatment, and then simply relaxing while the therapy takes place.

c) Once the treatment has finished, any excess gel that hasn't been absorbed into your skin can be washed off with warm water/mild soap and a cloth.

How Long Does a Treatment Last?

The length of time for each session will vary depending on which part of the body is being treated, however, as a guide, most sessions will last between 20 and 30 minutes.

Who is the Treatment For?

Red light therapy can treat various ailments either on its own or in conjunction with other types of treatment, medication, physiotherapy, or surgery.

RLT can be used for: -

- pain relief
- sports injuries

- anti-inflammatory effects
- skin conditions such as psoriasis and eczema
- scarring, including stretch marks
- muscle or joint problems, such as a sprained ankle or golf/tennis elbow
- cosmetic purposes

What Should I Expect from My First Treatment?

Most likely, your therapist will fully explain what constitutes the treatment and what you should expect from it, but they should also ask if <u>you</u> have any questions about the treatment itself or your treatment plan in general.

It's essential to get all the facts before agreeing to treatment, so it's advisable not to be shy about asking anything in connection with something that isn't clear to you or is bothering you.

If red light therapy is used for cosmetic purposes, it will most likely be applied to the face, in which case cream or a gel may be applied before treatment begins, which, by way of using red light, is absorbed into the skin. This should not cause any adverse effects and as long as you stick to the recommended number of treatments, you shouldn't have any problems.

However, if you are being treated for another reason that requires the light to be applied close to your eyes or over a large area of your face, make sure that all safety procedures are understood, in place, and correctly followed.

Because this type of treatment can be used for anti-ageing purposes, the patient's skin must be carefully monitored at all times during a session and series of sessions.

Skin Rejuvenation with Red Light Therapy

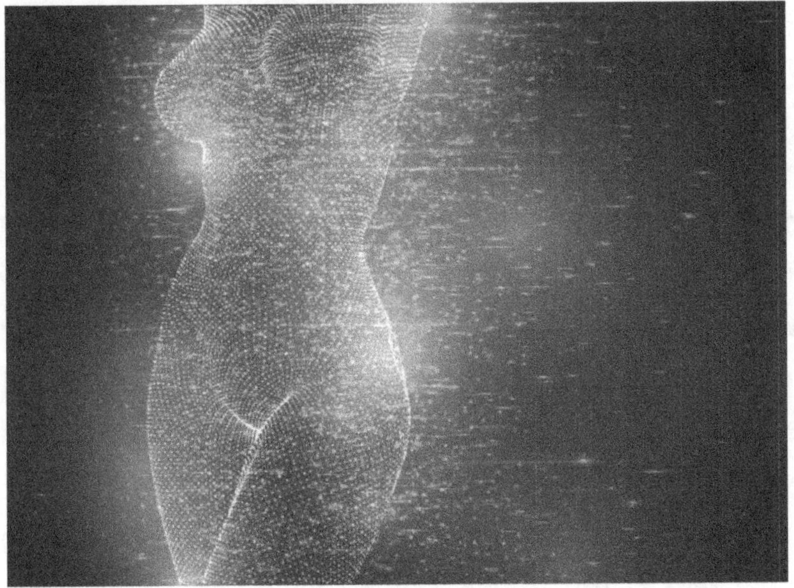

Skin conditions are among the most prevalent of all diseases and afflictions. It is estimated that over half of people in the Western world have some form of skin disorder, from minor irritations to life-threatening conditions like cancer.

Luckily, a significant amount of research has been conducted on how red light therapy can treat various skin ailments.

Mild Conditions

Red light therapy can be very effective in dealing with minor skin conditions. For one of the more common afflictions, acne, RLT is one of the first things many medical professionals turn to.

According to studies, red light regularly produces positive results in treating acne and can even prevent its return in people who had not seen relief from their symptoms before.

What makes red light so effective for treating acne is that it has a positive effect on inhibiting P. acnes bacteria, which are significant factors in causing breakouts and inflamed skin.

It does this by reducing the proliferation of P. acnes in sebaceous glands. This reduces the oil, dead skin cells, and bacteria that contribute to clogged pores and, in turn, acne outbreaks.

Blisters & Wounds

Red light therapy can also be used to treat more severe skin conditions like blisters and wounds. Treating blisters with red light is effective because it not only offers pain relief, but also reduces the risk of further infection.

Studies have found that red light therapy can help treat blisters and other wounds in a matter of days, making it a much faster, more efficient methodology than typical treatment, which all too often merely constitutes leaving them to heal by themselves.

However, this is not saying that red light therapy should be considered an alternative to all forms of treatment for blisters and wounds.

For wounds, it should only be regarded as a possible treatment if the bleeding has already stopped or is under control.

Also, some injuries will not respond well to red light, and some may actually become irritated by RLT. This includes ulcers caused by poor circulation or peripheral vascular disease, and infected wounds, which are known to promote inflammation.

Very importantly, red light therapy helps prevent blisters from becoming infected because it kills off the very bacteria responsible for *causing* wound infections. According to a study, even using red light therapy after a blister has formed can reduce its size and disease risk by 70%.

Eczema

Red light therapy is also an effective treatment for eczema.

Eczema is common among people with allergies and skin conditions like acne, but it can also develop among people who have suffered from long-term use of corticosteroids. It is characterized by the development of red, itchy skin that can become infected with bacteria.

In recent years, studies have found that red light therapy can help to reduce inflammation while improving blood flow. As a result, this reduces the itching characteristic of eczema and prevents the skin from becoming damaged, reduces inflammation and pain, and even prevents cracking of the skin.

Psoriasis & Dermatitis

Red light has also been used to successfully treat common skin conditions like psoriasis and dermatitis. These conditions are characterized by skin inflammation that results in red, flaky, and scaly patches on the body.

Treating psoriasis with red light works because it can reduce the levels of keratinocytes in the outer layer of skin, reducing its build-up, and preventing it from accumulating into plaques.

The same goes for dermatitis. Red light therapy works by causing the release of cytokines, which are chemicals that influence skin regeneration and inflammation in response to trauma or injury. By increasing cytokine release, red light therapy speeds up skin regeneration to improve the appearance of dermatitis and prevent damage.

For these skin conditions, RLT works best when used in conjunction with other types of treatment, such as a topical steroid cream or ointment. Used in this way, it doesn't just help to reduce inflammation, but also allows the cream/ointment to be absorbed more quickly into the skin.

Cellulite

Red light therapy is also effective in treating cellulite because it helps to break down fat cells which can then be eliminated through the body's lymphatic system. This allows cellulite to be treated from both inside and outside the body, making the treatment more efficient than some other forms that cannot penetrate through to the deeper layers of skin, and can only work from the outside (e.g., creams etc.)

Red light therapy can also stimulate collagen production in the skin, which will improve the appearance of cellulite by reducing its "lumpy" nature and help prevent it from returning. The collagen produced during treatment will boost skin elasticity and firmness.

Anti-ageing

Red light therapy can also treat wrinkles and reduce the visibility of fine lines, age spots, and other blemishes that can appear as part of the ageing process. This is because red light stimulates fibroblast activity in the lower layers of the skin, which increases collagen production.

Collagen makes up the bulk of your skin's connective tissue and plays a vital role in maintaining skin elasticity.

When used at low energy levels, RLT increases blood flow, and by increasing blood flow to your face, red light therapy promotes the growth of new skin cells and helps the body remove waste products that accumulate in the lower layers of skin.
In addition, by increasing blood flow, RLT can also promote tissue regeneration, reduce inflammation caused by sun damage, and promote the growth of elastin.

Along with collagen, elastin is a protein responsible for maintaining skin elasticity, therefore stimulating its production can help to improve the appearance of the skin.

Red light therapy is particularly effective at fighting the signs of ageing around the eyes and mouth. This is because the skin tissues in these areas are thinner and contain fewer blood vessels and, by virtue, less blood, making them more responsive to red light therapy.

Hair Loss and Therapy

Red light therapy has been used as an alternative option for hair loss. Frequently, hair loss can be due to various illnesses or side effects from certain medications. However, there are also cases where the cause is unknown, and sometimes, though obviously not always, treatment with red light therapy can help.

Loss of hair can be due to several different reasons, including endocrine, genetic, inflammatory, and infectious causes for hair loss in both men and women.

Red light therapy has been used to treat an autoimmune condition known as alopecia areata in which the body's immune system attacks the hair follicles. This condition affects over 2 million people worldwide.

In other cases, hair loss can be caused by an internal or external stressor to the body, such as a nutritional deficiency. For example, Vitamin B12 is essential in maintaining healthy blood flow to the scalp and follicles, and a deficiency can have a negative impact. Dihydrotestosterone (DHT) has a significant influence in male pattern baldness. DHT binds to receptors in sensitive cells within the hair follicle, which in turn recruits immune cells that have the unwanted effect of damaging and shrinking the affected partition.

Red light therapy has been found effective at inhibiting the production of this hormone and reducing the inflammation associated with it.

This combination of factors makes red light therapy a worthwhile course of action in men suffering from alopecia areata, even though results are, obviously, far from universal and are definitely not guaranteed.

Even though it may not work at all, because of the relatively low cost and ease of treatment, some people feel it's at least worth a try.

In addition, stem cells in the hair follicles are activated when exposed to red light therapy. This has stimulated hair growth in some individuals, even after completing other treatments for their condition.

It has been found that RLT is best used in conjunction with other therapies such as Minoxidil and Finasteride, both of which inhibit DHT production, more so than using either treatment alone.

In addition, combining these two therapies means that lower doses than is typically required for each treatment can be used, resulting in fewer side effects than is sometimes associated with higher dosages.

As well as treating alopecia areata and hair loss caused by dihydrotestosterone, red light therapy has also been shown to sometimes help restore hair growth in women with female pattern baldness who are suffering from low estrogen levels after menopause.

The process here is the same: red light stimulates stem cell activity, resulting in healthier follicles that produce thicker and more nourished hair strands.

In some hair loss cases, red light therapy's effectiveness is because it can help both men and women restore natural testosterone levels in their bodies.

(N.B. There is a general misconception that only men produce testosterone and only women produce estrogen, but in reality, both sexes produce both hormones, it's just that they produce them at different levels and ratios).

This allows the endocrine system to balance itself once again, which helps reduce the effects associated with alopecia areata, male pattern baldness, and female pattern baldness.

Musculoskeletal Conditions and Red Light Therapy

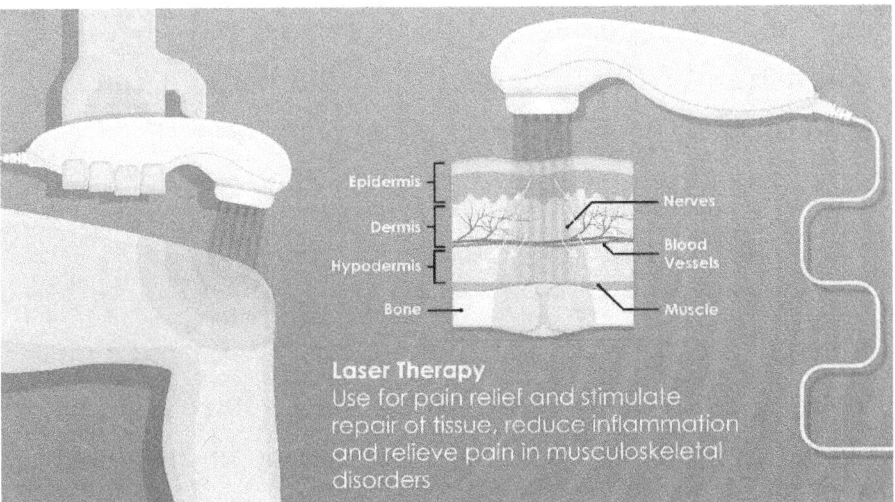

One of the most common uses for red light therapy is treating musculoskeletal conditions. These are a group of diseases that affect our body's bones, muscles, and joints. Because these are all systems of our body that work together, what affects one can, and very often does, also affect another or several other parts at once.

Many people have successfully used red light therapy for these conditions because of the potent anti-inflammatory and antioxidant effects.

RLT can be used alone or in conjunction with another treatment like acupuncture, chiropractic care, or even massage therapy. The light used provides wavelengths that help promote cell and tissue repair, and since it's non-harmful (if used correctly) to the body, it can be used practically anywhere.

Joint Pain

Joint pain can be helped tremendously with red light therapy, whether it's a knee injury in a runner that has persisted for months, arthritis pain from an old injury that pops up unexpectedly like sciatica, or chronic hip and back pain from sitting down too much at work.

Stiffness and Swelling

Reducing swelling and inflammation around joints using red light therapy helps lower stiffness and discomfort. Since swelling causes pain in the first place, it makes sense that you will experience less discomfort if you treat the swelling.

Reduce pain and discomfort

Red light therapy can help reduce pain and discomfort in many types of conditions, whether it's due to old injuries, inflammation, or arthritis. Because it's a natural way to treat the body, with no drugs or surgery required, many people opt to try RLT as a "first port of call".

Muscle Strain

Muscle strain from an injury, like those you can easily pick up from sports, is expected when you're active, it's par for the course (pun entirely intended!).

Regardless of what activity you do that brought about the muscle strain, whether it's running, weight lifting, or even gardening, red light therapy can provide relief. It helps the muscle to heal faster and is certainly more efficient than simply waiting for it to heal on its own without treatment.

This is achieved by increasing blood flow to the damaged area, which helps deliver more nutrients than usual, thus significantly speeding up the recovery process.

Bone Injury

Bone injuries can be painful and slow to heal, depending on the severity and location in the body. These injuries have a very high rate of infection complications because bones are porous and provide an area for bacteria to linger if not appropriately cleaned or treated quickly with antibiotics.

Because red light therapy increases circulation throughout your body, it's been shown effective for treating bone infections when used in conjunction with antibiotics like penicillin.

Cell Repair

Red light therapy is well known to speed up cell repair. RLT can help with the rehabilitation of ligaments and tendons, such as those in the knees, ankles, back, elbows, shoulders, and wrists.

Because of the deep penetration of red light therapy, it can be used for <u>any</u> muscle pain, or inflammation anywhere in the body - even those that reside more deeply, like a rotator cuff injury, for example.

There are many more uses for RLT in connection with musculoskeletal conditions, but these are just some of the more common ones.

Medical Benefits of Red Light Therapy

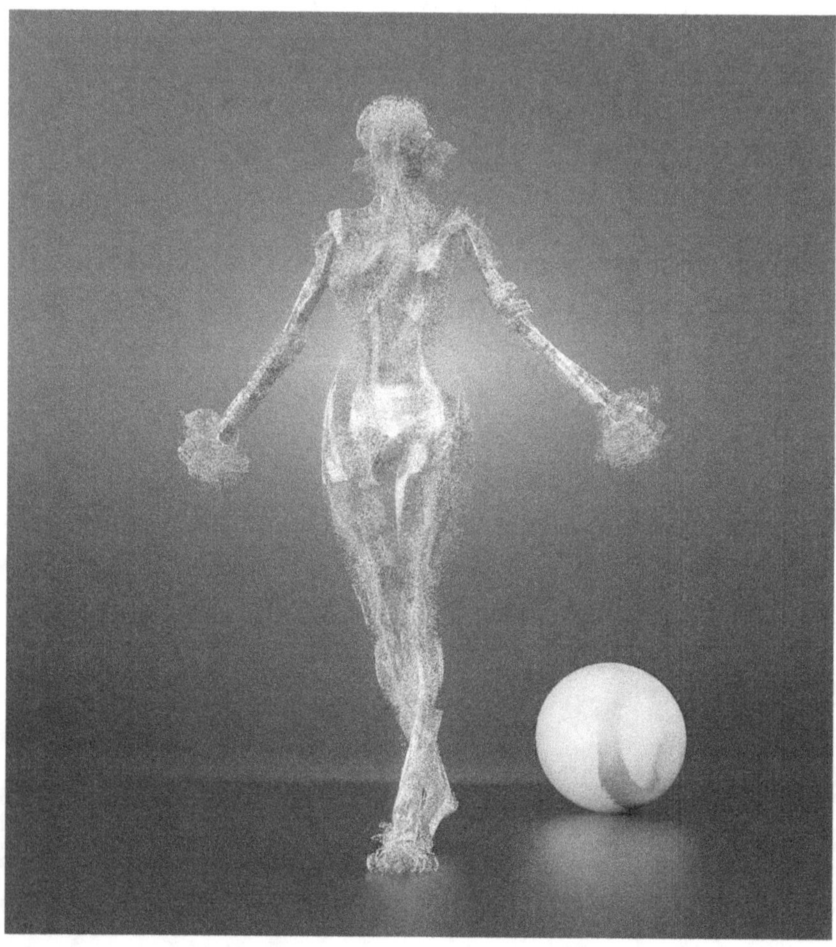

As already stated, many different medical conditions can benefit from red light therapy. However, it is essential to note that while the treatments are generally safe and effective for most people, they should not be used as a substitute for standard medical care being administered by a licensed doctor or therapist.

Any individual suffering from an illness should always consult with their physician before using red light therapy.

As with all procedures, red light therapy does not guarantee any cure, but it may help alleviate certain symptoms and positively impact several ailments.

Inflammation

Chronic inflammation is undoubtedly the root cause of the majority of today's health problems.

R.L.T. can reduce inflammation by inducing hyperoxygenation of the blood cells, thus optimizing circulation, improving immune response, and reducing the stress response, which is itself a cause of inflammation.

Infrared light also increases ATP energy production, higher levels of which have been found to be linked to lower levels of inflammation.

Just to emphasise how damaging inflammation is, it is a major contributory factor for disease in the following areas of the body:

- Brain
- Liver
- Skin
- Thyroid
- Cardiovascular
- Lungs
- GI Tract
- Bones/Joints
- Kidneys

Arthritis Relief

Arthritis involves inflammation developing in joints which, in turn, leads to pain and stiffness. Red light stimulates the mitochondria within cells which are involved in producing energy, and this results in reducing inflammation associated with arthritis, especially rheumatoid arthritis.

Additionally, collagen production is stimulated, which results in making the joints more flexible. Poor blood circulation to muscles and joints reduces the amount of oxygen available for cellular activity, resulting in pain and stiffness.

Red light therapy increases blood flow to both muscles and joints, resulting in reduced discomfort.

Gastrointestinal Disorders

Red light has a calming effect on gastric muscles, which can help gut disorders such as IBS (Irritable Bowel Syndrome).

The therapy increases the amount of serotonin in the digestive tract, which results in enhancing intestinal motility.

Additionally, the anti-inflammatory properties of red light reduce inflammation in the bowels and stimulate the digestive system.

Red light also stimulates the mucous membranes within the intestinal walls which means they "replenish" themselves faster and prevent leaky gut syndrome.

Additionally, red light helps alleviate bacterial imbalance which is a common cause of gastrointestinal upset.

Detoxification

Red light therapy helps with general body detoxification by way of the following processes:

- Increases blood flow
- Stimulates the lymphatic system
- Reduces inflammation
- Stimulates cell mitochondria
- Reduces cellulite
- Stabilising circadian rhythms
- Clears toxins from the skin
- Increases ATP production
- Stimulates cell repair

This happens by way of general detoxification and is not necessarily dependent upon where the infrared light is applied. In other words, you can treat one area of the body with RLT and experience benefits in other areas. This process is known as "remote tissue conditioning".

Boosting Immunity

In addition to alleviating symptoms associated with autoimmune diseases, red light therapy can help enhance immunity by increasing natural killer cells (NK) and cytokine production.

Researchers have also discovered that low amounts of red light therapy can boost white blood cell production and lead to better plasma volume, lymphocyte, neutrophil, and basophil counts.

Reducing inflammation also improves immune function and so protects against bacterial and viral infections.

Additionally, when lymphatic vessels are flooded with blood from increased circulation, it removes toxins more effectively from joint spaces and muscles where they reside, resulting in reduced pain.

Weight Loss, Fat Loss and Obesity

Red light therapy not only stimulates your metabolism, resulting in weight loss, but it also breaks down body fat. It does so by inhibiting the production and release of cortisol, a stress hormone that has been linked to weight gain.

Additionally, it stimulates the lymphatic system and reduces inflammation resulting in better blood circulation and breakdown of stored fat.

Not only does RLT break down existing body fat, it can prevent the future accumulation of new fat cells, so a real win-win!

Studies have shown it does this by increasing adiponectin levels which results in not only burning more calories, but also in decreasing appetite. Given that we tend to eat more when stressed or anxious, reducing stress through RLT can be a real benefit.

Cancer

There is conflicting evidence and contradictory opinions as to the effectiveness of RLT in connection with cancer.

Some studies seem to find beneficial effects, while others appear to find the opposite and that it can actually make the condition worse and possibly lead to an increase in the number of cancer cells/size of tumor.

However, it is known that red light therapy can help reduce inflammation and swelling, and this means that it can help manage side effects like lymphedema (fluid retention), edema, gastrointestinal problems including mouth sores and esophagitis, fever, or chills - all of which are usually related to chemotherapy.

This being the case, the author encourages the reader to neither embrace nor dismiss the possibility of using RLT in conjunction with any form of cancer treatment without doing their own research and, most definitely, without first discussing it with their doctor/consultant/health care provider.

To help, here are two links to articles that I think are of interest: -

1) thepaleomom.com/red-light-therapy-for-cancer/

2) cancer.gov/about-cancer/treatment/types/photoimmunity-video

Photoimmunotherapy

Photoimmunotherapy is a brand-new kind of cancer therapy involving near-infrared light (NIRL) which utilizes an antibody to which a photoabsorbing chemical is connected that is sensitive to/triggered by NIRL.

How it works:

The antibody-photoabsorber conjugate (Antibody Drug Conjugates or ADCs) are special drugs that combine antibodies specific to the surface antigens that are on tumor cells with potent anti-cancer agents, both of which are combined via a chemical linker) is injected into the person receiving treatment, which then travels through the bloodstream to eventually reach the tumor itself where it binds to unique receptors on the surface of the cancer cells.

As soon as the conjugate is bound to cancer cells, the photoabsorbing chemical can be triggered by using near-infrared light.

When the chemical has been triggered, it causes instant damage to the cell membrane making it possible for water that is outside of the cell to now enter it, causing the cell to swell. (Close-by cells without the special receptors will not be affected.)

Increased pressure within the swollen cell eventually causes the membrane to burst and die, a process known as necrosis.

This cell necrosis causes the tumor to shrink in size and will eventually disappear with healthy tissue regrowing in its place.

Photoimmunotherapy is a new kind of cancer therapy that is extremely specific for cancer cells and does not damage nearby typical cells.

It is presently in clinical trials in patients with inoperable growths.

Reduce High Blood Pressure

An increase in blood flow due to red light therapy helps lower high blood pressure while simultaneously strengthening the endothelial tissue lining in blood vessels leading to improved cardiovascular health.

Additionally, red light therapy has been shown to reduce arterial stiffness in blood vessels, which is another way that it helps to bring blood pressure down.

Athletic Recovery

Many athletes use red light therapy as a form of recovery immediately after a workout or competition in order to reduce muscle pain and speed up recovery and healing time. This is especially important for individuals who use heavy weights while training for strength and endurance, which can cause muscle micro-tears.

RLT does this by increasing blood flow to muscles, reducing inflammation, preventing free radical damage, and stimulating collagen production within muscles, which results in faster recovery times and a reduced likelihood of injury.

Pain Management

Red light therapy can be effective in pain management for several reasons.

Firstly, inflammation is one of the most common triggers linked with pain, especially in arthritis sufferers, and, as stated, red light therapy reduces inflammation, thus resulting in reduced, or sometimes even eliminated, pain.

Additionally, it increases blood circulation, allowing oxygen and nutrients to reach damaged tissues more effectively, meaning cells heal faster.

Interestingly, RLT has been shown to reduce the frequency and severity of migraine headaches by stimulating serotonin release within the brain stem area and by increasing serotonin receptors in the thalamus area.

The physical process by which RLT helps in pain management, reduction, or elimination is by way of the stimulation and production of endorphins and neurotransmitters, which are natural painkillers produced within the body.

Endorphins are released when you exercise, and this release of endorphins acts on opioid receptors, resulting in less intense pain signals being transmitted to the brain.

Similarly, activating certain neurotransmitters can also produce analgesic effects that reduce pain sensitivity by inhibiting neuron firing and swelling around injured or inflamed tissues.

Role of Red Light Therapy in Mental Health

In the previous chapter, it detailed how red light therapy can be used for healing physical issues. However, its uses go beyond only physical applications.

This chapter describes its role in alleviating mental health conditions using specific wavelengths of red light.

The following are some of the mental health issues and disorders that have shown promising results when using red light therapy:

Seasonal Affective Disorder

Seasonal Affective Disorder (SAD) is a type of depression triggered by exposure to seasonal changes such as fewer daylight hours, or even heavy rainfall. In these cases, RLT can be an effective treatment option.

The administration of red light therapy for a ten week period has been shown to improve symptoms in people suffering from SAD.

RLT affects the body's circadian rhythm, which in turn can have a direct influence on mood. As such, it can sometimes be an effective treatment for seasonal major depressive disorder (S-MDD) or seasonal bipolar disorder (S-BPD).

Depression

Red light therapy has been found to be effective in treating patients with depression and other mental health conditions.

In one study, the patients were divided into two groups. One group was exposed to red light therapy, while the other received a placebo treatment.

The results showed that most of those who used red light therapy experienced significant improvement in their condition compared to the placebo group.

This is because depression is sometimes considered an illness that can be caused by serotonin depletion. Red light exposure leads to increased synthesis of serotonin – a vital neurotransmitter associated with good mental health - thus helping to alleviate depression.

A note of caution, however. One possible side effect of using this therapy is the worsening depressive symptoms in patients with bipolar disorder (note: this is different to *seasonal* bi-polar disorder).

Light is known to alter serotonin production, and people suffering from mood disorders are characteristically sensitive to changes in their serotonin levels, which can, in turn, lead to manic or hypomanic episodes.

By stimulating the head area either directly or remotely (i.e. applying the NIR light to other areas of the body) areas of the brain linked to certain types of depression and anxiety are activated, in particular, dlPFC and vmPFC, and this leads to a reduction in the severity of the symptoms.

In a small study of 10 people, all of whom had major depression and 9 of which also had anxiety, RLT was used to monitor its effectiveness to treat these disorders.

After only 2 weeks, 6 patients showed improvement in depression symptoms and 7 patients showed improvement in anxiety symptoms.

There were no side effects reported.

Anxiety

Numerous studies have shown that RLT can produce excellent results when treating anxiety.

Anxiety is a very common but nonetheless debilitating mental health condition. In fact, according to the Anxiety and Depression Center of America, "Anxiety disorders are the most common mental illness in the United States, affecting 40 million adults every year."

You would almost expect that in order to experience benefit from red light therapy when the condition being treated is that of an emotional or psychological origin that you might have to apply the light straight to the head, but this is not the case, although direct cranial application is an option and does produce excellent results.

This is because RLT is known to increase the efficiency of mitochondria and there are free-roaming mitochondria circulating in our bloodstream, so those mitochondria that have been energised by the red and near-infrared light can journey to other locations in the body in order to transfer their energy to where it is needed.

In other words, you can treat one area of the body with RLT and experience benefits in other areas due to a process known as "remote tissue conditioning".

Also, treating the gut area with RLT will have a very positive effect on the patient's mental state because it is now known that there is a direct connection between the gut and the brain via the vagus nerve.

In addition, a great deal of the body's serotonin is produced in the gut and serotonin levels are dramatically linked to, and are directly responsible for, mood and anxiety control. The more your serotonin levels drop, the greater the level of anxiety and depression. So restoring gut health greatly helps to restore mental health.

Another study was done with 15 patients suffering from Generalized Anxiety Disorder (GAD), the study lasting 8 weeks. They were exposed to Near Infrared Light (NIR) by using a red light therapy headband placed on the patient's forehead. Base tests were conducted before and after the treatment and there was a significant improvement in all GAD symptoms in all patients.

Attention Deficit Disorder and Attention Deficit Hyperactivity Disorder

Red light therapy has been shown to improve the cognitive abilities of people with Attention Deficit Disorder (ADD) and Attention Deficit Hyperactivity Disorder (ADHD).

However, no studies point to specific wavelengths of light that should be used for treating this mental health disorder.

ADHD and ADD are often caused by a deficiency of specific neurotransmitters such as dopamine. When exposed to red light, the specific areas that regulate mood and cognition stimulate the release of dopamine, serotonin, and norepinephrine – all of which are neurotransmitters associated with cognitive abilities.

As a point of interest, it is believed that these neurotransmitters can also be depleted by stress and lack of sleep, the latter of which being of particular concern when individuals of a certain age group very often stay up late playing online games, streaming, or engaging in other internet-based activities.

As a double whammy, the blue light emitted by devices is known to interfere with the levels of specific hormones that are crucial to deep, restorative sleep, meaning that what little sleep the individual gets is of very poor quality.

PTSD (Post-Traumatic Stress Disorder)

Exposure to red light slows the production of cortisol, which is a hormone associated with stress and fear. This, in turn, relieves symptoms of PTSD such as anxiety, panic attacks, and avoidance behavior.

Some treatments for PTSD involve exposure to light that is rich in blue wavelengths. However, this may harm memory and cognition.

Red light therapy stimulates the release of neurotransmitters such as serotonin, which calms the patient, thus reducing their stress levels. It is also believed to improve sleep patterns, leading to improvement in the patient's overall mental health.

Interestingly, memory performance can be improved by exposing yourself to bright light between one and two hours after waking up in the morning. Since cortisol levels fall after two hours of wakefulness, it is assumed that this is the time when your brain cells are open to stimulation by bright light.

In comparison to blue light, red light does not affect cortisol levels as much and, as such, can be used at any time of day without having to worry about it affecting your circadian rhythm.

How to Conduct Red Light Therapy at Home

There are specific methods with which to conduct red light therapy at home and many of these resources are readily available on the internet. However, before you spend money on any of them, it is essential that you understand your specific requirements, and purchase a suitable product accordingly.

If you do want to purchase equipment for conducting red light therapy, keep the following points in mind:

1) Always go for the highest power LED or full-spectrum bulb available (the intensity should be specified on the label); it should emit at least 90-100 lumens/watts.
   This is because when you are using the equipment for an extended period of weeks and months, the intensity of light will remain consistent throughout, whereas if you purchase a low-power unit, then after a few months it could start to get dimmer. Obviously, it's better to invest in a unit that gives consistent bright light even after many months of usage.

2) Always try to purchase equipment that's been approved by the FDA or other international agencies; this will give you confidence in the knowledge that whatever product you are buying is indeed effective and will help you get the desired results.

3) It is advisable to purchase a lamp that does not have any color filters because it is better to get treatment without any particular color wavelength being interrupted. If you want professional results, it might be best to go for near-infrared panels

If you wish to conduct red light therapy in the comfort of your own home, follow these steps:

1) Firstly, be sure to read the manual provided with the product in its entirety. It will guide you through how to use, install, and maintain the equipment properly.

   Most people are sometimes guilty of "skim-reading" instruction manuals (me included!), but as this is a procedure that affects your body and health, in this case it's definitely worth the time invested.

Generally, it only takes a few minutes to set up any equipment that's designed for conducting red light therapy at home.

2) Place an LED lamp on one side of your room (near any window) so that it can deliver light to your entire body.

3) Then close the doors and windows of your room and turn it on; make sure that there is no sunlight or any kind of external light entering your room during therapy sessions.

4) One of the more essential things in red light therapy is "duration"; you must spend at least 20 minutes daily under red lights for the best possible results.

Some people report that after spending time under these lights, they feel quite fatigued and lethargic. If this happens, stop treatment for a few days and resume only when you start feeling fresh again (this is generally within a week).

The use of red light therapy is increasing day by day because it can provide several health benefits, yet without affecting any other part of the body.

As long as LED therapy lamps are used correctly, they could prove to be beneficial and time well spent.

The Do and Don't of At Home Treatment with Red Light Therapy

As with any other medication or treatment, you must be aware of the dos and don'ts in order to achieve the desired results.

The following discusses some of the more important points you need to remember during red light therapy.

Do:

i)   It is essential to understand that the effects of red light therapy are only achieved when you spend at least 20 minutes daily under the lamps, though not necessarily all in one sitting.

Duration may vary from person to person, and be dependent on the condition being treated, ***but always read the manufacturer's instructions and guidelines.***

ii)   Spending a minimum of 7-8 hours in darkness (absolute darkness) during the night ensures better results.

Don't:

i) Avoid using moisturizers or any oil on the treated area because the oily top layers of skin will absorb much of the light, possibly resulting in red light not penetrating to the deeper layers.

ii) Avoid drinking and smoking during red light therapy sessions as this might affect the body's blood circulation and lead to side effects.

iii) Avoid eating anything 1 hour before treatment.

iv) If you experience any itching, redness, or rashes on the skin while conducting red light therapy sessions, discontinue treatment and consult your doctor immediately.

Side Effects of Red Light Therapy

Red light therapy, like most alternative medicine therapies, has a low risk of side effects. Research suggests that only two percent of people who have used red light therapy have reported adverse reactions or side effects.

Discomfort During Treatment

The intensity of the red light may cause some discomfort to those with sensitive skin or more acute conditions. The use of topical analgesics eases this discomfort. If you feel any unusual pain during treatment, stop using the device and consult a doctor immediately.

Excessive Use

It is not recommended to use red light therapy for more than 10 - 20 minutes per treatment. In case of excessive exposure (i.e., longer than 20 minutes), your body may suffer from a sunburn-like reaction, which can negatively affect the skin. While regular sessions are encouraged, it's important to avoid long sittings.

Theoretically, there is no set limit with red light therapy devices. However, excessive application might result in nausea or dizziness due to overstimulation of the immune system, or the "heating up" of tissues deep inside the body to a level of that beyond the normal core temperature.

As with many other therapies and medications, it is advisable to consult your doctor before using RLT devices. This can help you gain a better understanding of the complete procedure and the potential side effects.

Mild Side Effects

At times, red light therapy can result in mild side effects. These usually disappear as the body gets used to the treatment, but you may want to take note of these in case they persist or aggravate:

- Headache
- Tiredness
- Nausea
- Muscle pain

If you experience any of them at any level, stop using the device and visit your doctor immediately for advice.

Rarely do patients need medication because such side effects are not usually serious, unless you develop an allergy or hypersensitivity that requires immediate medical attention.

If there is more than negligible discomfort, it's important to discontinue use and consult a doctor to monitor your condition if necessary and decide on future treatments.

People who have heart disease, depression, or are pregnant should not use red light therapy unless under strict supervision.

Common Side Effects

The most common side effects are feelings of warmth or tingling on the skin surface where light was applied. These should pass within a short time of completement of treatment and turning off the lamp unit, as long as there is no actual injury to your body tissue due to heat build-up in the area exposed to red light.

If you experience any of the following after using the device, stop treatment and consult your doctor:

- Skin discomfort or sensitivity
- Rash
- Itchiness
- Fever
- Severe headache

Get immediate medical help if your skin becomes very hot and forms blisters within a short period (minutes) after application.

This could be a sign of an overload reaction to the therapy and may require medication.

Some may even develop heart palpitations, so again, seek professional advice as soon as possible if this happens after using your device.

A doctor might monitor your condition for some time before administering red light therapy again, or even suggest an alternative treatment.

Who Should <u>Not</u> Undergo Red Light Therapy?

Red light therapy is generally safe, but certain individuals should avoid it.

The following is advice on who should not undergo red light therapy and gives information on contraindications.

a) Those with active skin cancer or precancerous lesions on the skin; this includes people with melanoma, actinic keratosis, and basal cell carcinoma.

b) It is also contraindicated for use by those who have photosensitive disorders like lupus erythematosus or lichen planus since these conditions can be exacerbated by exposure to red light.

c) People with light sensitivity of the retina (retinitis pigmentosa) could be worsened during treatment.

d) Individuals with active herpes simplex lesions in the area to be treated.

e) Pregnant women should not undergo red light therapy.

If you fall into one of the high-risk categories, consult your doctor before undergoing any treatment.

Certain drugs may cause unsafe phototoxic or photoallergic reactions with red light therapy. This includes oral contraceptives, tetracycline antibiotics, and diuretics, so always ask your doctor about possible contraindications <u>before</u> use of red light therapy.

Red Light Therapy vs Infrared Saunas

Many people ask what the difference is between red light therapy and infrared saunas and the answer is very simple.

Infrared saunas use heat in order to be effective, whereas red light therapy emits almost no heat whatsoever.

Red and near-infrared wavelengths, which penetrate your cells, stimulate your mitochondria without necessitating the use of heat.

This is an important factor as these wavelengths give your cells energy and help eliminate inflammation without putting undue stress on your cardiovascular system.

Most users of infrared saunas report similar benefits to those associated with traditional saunas, and the majority of these benefits come from increased cardiovascular function caused by the heat.

They include:

- Relief from insomnia
- Relaxation
- Improved detoxification
- Reduced inflammation
- Weight loss
- Reduced muscle pain and soreness
- Decreased joint pain
- Improved circulation
- Relief from chronic fatigue syndrome
- Reduced insulin sensitivity
- Increased autophagy
- Increased production of growth hormone
- Improved immune response

Because of the above benefits associated with infrared saunas, it is definitely worth looking at using them as well as using red light therapy.

As is always the case, you must check with your doctor or professional health care provider before using any infrared saunas.

Which Other Therapies Can Be Used Best with Red Light?

We have already seen how red light therapy can be used in conjunction with other treatments and the following are further therapies that work best when combined with RLT.

Facial Rejuvenation

This therapy is highly effective when combined with red light as it provides deep penetration, in which the red light is essential for effective treatment.

A facial rejuvenation session will last between thirty and forty minutes to treat all the areas on and around the face. For best results, the combination of RLT and a facial rejuvenation session can be done two or three times a week.

Hair Restoration

This form of therapy involves red light and a topical solution, which is applied to the areas where hair loss has occurred before the treatment starts.

RLT irradiates photons into the dermal layers of the scalp tissues, and these photons are readily absorbed by weak cells which facilitates new hair growth.

Not only does the red light enable the topical solution to penetrate the skin's dermis layer, it also allows for better blood circulation which speeds up the hair growth.

A single treatment lasts thirty minutes and should be completed three times a week. In the majority of cases, hair regrowth is observed after 12 to 26 weeks.

It's generally accepted that the procedure is safe, and is certainly less invasive than undergoing transplant surgery.

Cellulite Treatment

To reduce cellulite build-up, specific areas such as thighs, buttocks, and hips should be treated with red light therapy along with a massage.

Anti-Ageing Treatment

As previously explained, red light therapy can be used to treat wrinkles and fine lines, but in order to make the treatment more effective, you can use an antioxidant solution or cream that will penetrate the skin and add an extra element of protection against free radicals released during the treatment.

Relieving Muscle Soreness

Red light therapy can work wonders when it comes to muscle soreness after a workout.

Those into serious training probably already know about the benefits of cryotherapy and how ice packs work to reduce pain and inflammation in the muscles. Red light penetrates deep into the muscle and also helps with tissue regeneration which means faster recovery time!

Red Light Therapy and COVID-19

The leading cause of death from COVID-19 infection is due to an exaggerated host immune response, resulting in inflammation and cytokine storms in the lungs.

Photobiomodulation therapy, which involves exposure to red or infrared light, is a well-documented therapy that is already being used to treat a range of diseases which have underlying inflammatory conditions.

It has been found that exposure to infrared light in two 10-minute sessions per day leads to a marked reduction in the inflammatory response pathway, which itself has been linked to the onset of the well-publicised cytokine storms in COVID-19 patients.

It's thought that, after undergoing red light therapy, a particular cellular mechanism may be activated which downregulates the host's immune response, leading to a decrease in inflammation.

The use of red light therapy in connection with the treatment of COVID-19 has been researched by studying its effectiveness along three fundamentally different applications.

Before I go any further it must be emphasized that at the time of going to publication these trials were still ongoing and in a relatively early research phase, but nonetheless showed initial promise.

As such the author recommends that if you are unfortunate enough to contract COVID, that you speak with your personal physician or the person assigned to specifically treat your COVID case as to the possible use of red light therapy.

Do not take it upon yourself to administer this therapy as a treatment for COVID-19 as the decision of whether or not to use RLT is one that must be made by a medical professional.

RLT Usage Method 1

The first possible use of red light therapy in the treatment of COVID-19 is by way of using light sources inserted into each nostril.

Studies have been done using this method whereby the level of virus present in the nasal cavity is measured both before and after treatment and it was found that there was a reduction in the level of virus after treatment with red light therapy.

The theory behind this treatment is that very often COVID-19 will enter the body via the nasal cavities due to the inhalation of the airborn virus (known as aerosol virus) which will then pass into the lungs causing the classic COVID-19 breathing difficulties.

So, it is surmised that if the virus can be eliminated in the initial stages "at source" in the nasal cavities before it spreads to the lungs, that this could be of great benefit.

Two caveats to this being that, as already stated, these are ongoing trials that need larger and further study, and, secondly, will only be effective in the very early stages of infection.

RLT Usage Method 2

The second possible use of red light therapy in the treatment of COVID-19 is by way of directly applying the light to the front and/or back of the thorax of the patient so as to specifically target the lungs in the hope that there will be a subsequent reduction in inflammation in the tissues and general structures of the lungs.

In one particular case, a patient received four consecutive sessions administered once daily of Near Infrared Light over the posterior chest area. Evaluation protocols such as x-rays and blood markers were taken both before and after the sessions.

Following RLT, the patient showed improvement in specific respiratory indicators such as radiological findings and inflammatory markers.

The results suggested that red light therapy in adjunct with COVID-19 treatment can potentially improve a patient's condition and general outcome and possibly negate the need for ventilator support and ICU admission, which, it has to be said, was initially expected for this particular patient.

However, there is always the possibility that this patient would have experienced the same improvement and outcome if the original COVID-19 treatment protocol was all that they received, which is why further and larger studies are also needed for this use of RLT.

RLT Usage Method 3

It was found that some COVID-19 patients accumulated a harmful level of iron in their blood. This was causing an intense system-wide inflammatory response with the consequence of increased C-reactive protein and albumin.

In the study, red and near-infrared radiation was administered (along with vitamin D using ultraviolet B radiation), to increase the production of Adenosine Triphosphate (ATP).

This seems to help with COVID-19 in two distinct ways:

Firstly, it is thought that due to photon absorption by way of the RLT, the stability of the iron in the blood increases, thus preventing the loss of its oxygen transportation function.

Secondly, RLT seems to regulate enzyme activity leading to a significant increase in the rate of oxygen consumption by mitochondria, thus increasing ATP production.

With COVID-19 being such an easily transmissible virus, which lead to the announcement by the World Health Organisation of a pandemic in March 2020, any treatment that shows either potential for, or a definite improvement of, patient outcome is worth further investigation, and this seems to be the case with red light therapy.

However, at the risk of sounding over-cautious or of re-stating the obvious, any thoughts of using RLT *must* be discussed with your professional healthcare provider in advance of potential treatment.

Final Thoughts

So, is Red Light Therapy a kind of magic, the panacea to cure all ills?

No… because no treatment is!

However, the science and studies behind red light therapy *is* incredibly promising.

There are several things to consider when thinking about red light therapy:

- **Is RLT covered by my health insurance?**
  Red light therapy is not necessarily a covered treatment. Contact your health insurance company before seeking treatment.

- **How many treatments will I need?**
  You'll more than likely need ongoing treatments. This could potentially add up to a lot of time and money.

- **Will I achieve the desired results?**
  Everyone's body is different, so results can and will vary.

- **Do you trust the person providing the red light therapy?**
  OK, so tanning salon vs. a medical professional? That's a bit of a no-brainer, I know, but the qualifications of the person delivering your treatment are paramount. After all, this is a medical procedure.

- **Is red light therapy an appropriate treatment for my skin condition?**
  Consult your professional healthcare provider before opting for RLT

I sincerely hope that you've enjoyed reading this book and that you've gained valuable insight into red light therapy, and if you do go ahead and try it for yourself, that you have an enjoyable and successful experience with it.

I wish you health and happiness wherever you may go.

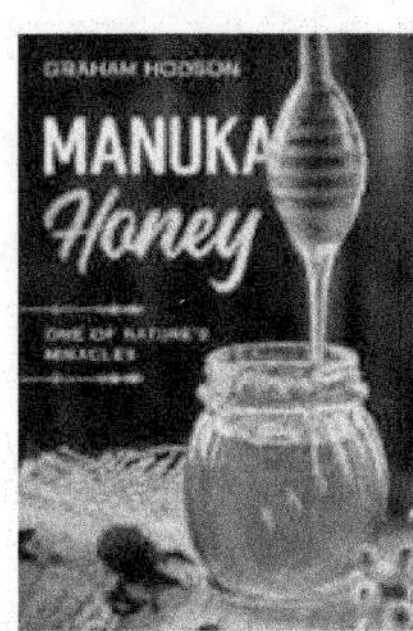

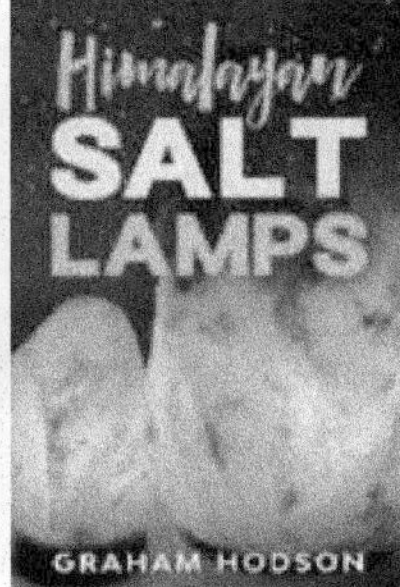

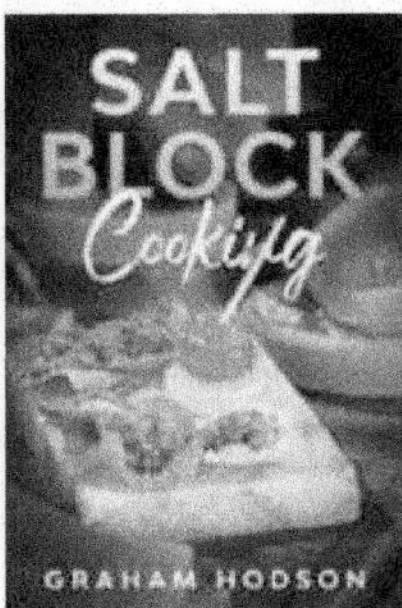

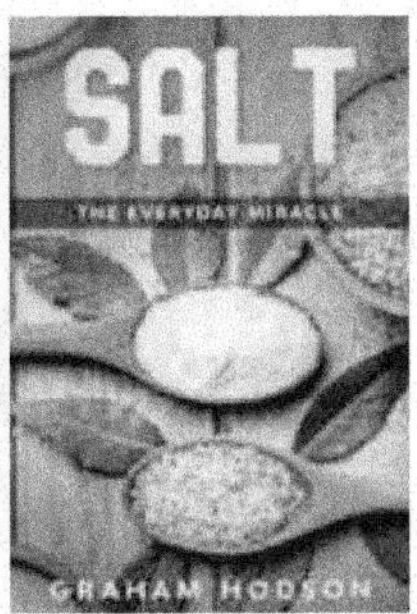

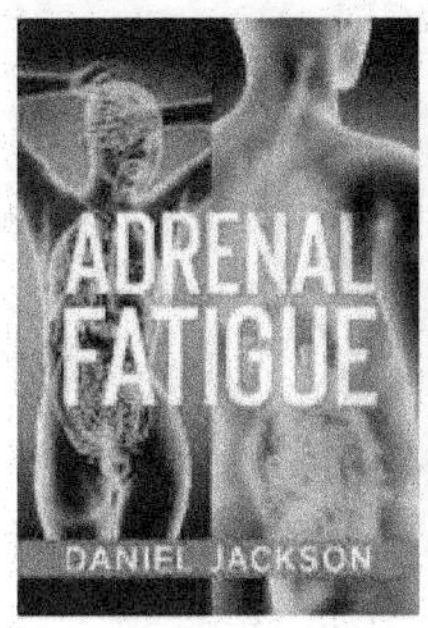

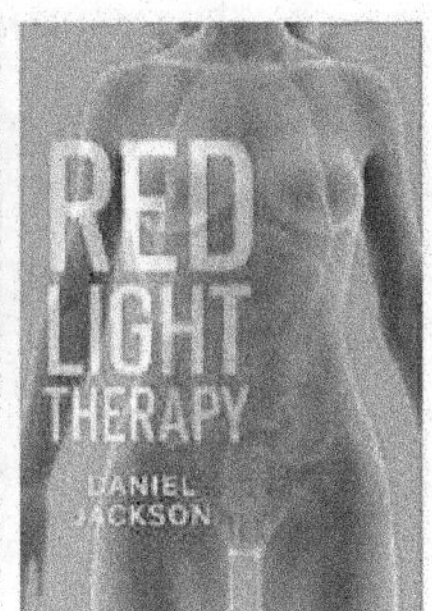

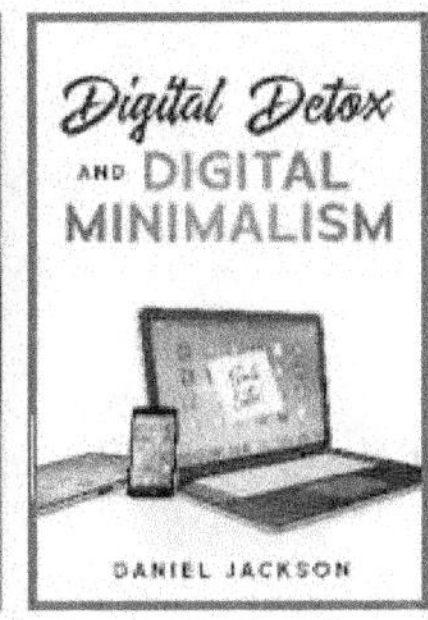

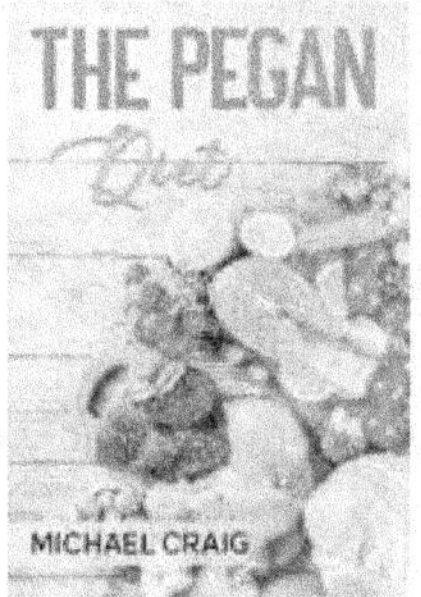

Take a look at more great books available from Rockwood Publishing

… some for FREE!

Just visit the link below:

rockwoodpublishing.co.uk

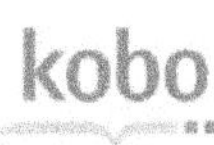
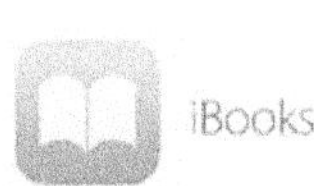

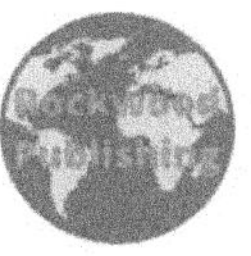

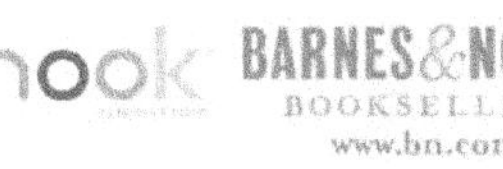

Index

publication, neither the author nor the affiliates assume any responsibility for errors, omissions or contrary interpretation of the subject matter herein. Any perceived slights to any specific person(s) or organisation(s) are purely unintentional. We have no control over the nature, content and availability of the websites listed in this book. The inclusion of any website links does not necessarily imply a recommendation or endorse the views expressed within them. Rockwood Publishing takes no responsibility for, and will not be liable for, the websites being temporarily unavailable or being removed from the Internet. The accuracy and completeness of information provided herein and opinions stated herein are not guaranteed or warranted to produce any particular results, and the advice and strategies contained herein may not be suitable for every individual. The author shall not be liable for any loss incurred as a consequence of the use and application, directly or indirectly, of any information presented in this work. This publication is designed to provide information in regards to the subject matter covered. The information included in this book has been compiled to give an overview of the subject(s) and detail some of the symptoms, treatments etc. that are available to people with this condition. It is not intended to give medical advice. For a firm diagnosis of your condition, and for a treatment plan suitable for you, you should consult your doctor or consultant. The writer of this book and the publisher are not responsible for any damages or negative consequences following any of the treatments or methods highlighted in this book. Website links are for informational purposes and should not be seen as a personal endorsement; the same applies to the products detailed in this book. The reader should also be aware that although the web links included were correct at the time of writing, they may become out of date in the future.

Disclaimers

The content contained within this book is for information and entertainment purposes only, and in no way purports to represent professional medical opinion. It should NOT be used as a substitute for expert advice, and you must consult with your designated health professional before acting upon any information contained herein or before undertaking any practice whose methodology is referred to in this book. The author is NOT a registered health professional and the text merely represents personal opinion, not medical fact. The author cannot be held responsible for the consequences of any action derived from the reading of this book, as the content is not based on diagnosis and subsequent regimen. It is the reader's responsibility to seek proper, professional medical advice from a registered health practitioner in connection with any material contained within this book.

Legal Disclaimer (part 1)

Nothing in this book should be construed as an attempt to diagnose, treat or cure. The information in this book is intended to be a community resource. The author takes no responsibility for any informational material or brochures produced using information taken from this book. The author has endeavoured to ensure that all information is correct at the time of publication. This information, however, is subject to change without notice. The author makes no warranty with regard to the accuracy of any information and will not be liable for any errors or omissions. Any liability that arises as a result of this information is hereby excluded to the fullest extent allowed by law.
This information should not be used as a substitute for seeking independent professional advice.

Legal Disclaimer (part 2)

Disclaimer and Terms of Use:

a) i. In publishing this information, the author makes no representations concerning the efficacy, appropriateness or suitability of any products or treatments. Use this information at your own risk. The compiler is not a doctor and has no medical background or training.

ii. Statements and information regarding dietary supplements, books and any products mentioned have not been evaluated by any health authority and are not intended to diagnose, treat, cure or prevent any disease or health condition.

b) In view of the possibility of human error, neither the author nor any other party involved in providing this information, warrant that the information contained therein is in every respect accurate or complete and they are not responsible nor liable for any errors or omissions that may be found or for the results obtained from the use of such information. The entire risk as to use of this information is assumed by the user.

c) You are encouraged to consult other sources and confirm the information.

d) The information you access is provided "as is". No warranty, expressed or implied, is given as to the accuracy, completeness or timeliness of any information herein, or for obtaining legal advice. To the fullest extent permissible pursuant to applicable law, neither the author nor any other parties who have been involved in the creation, preparation, printing, or delivering of this information assume responsibility for the completeness, accuracy, timeliness, errors or omissions of said information and assume no liability for any direct, incidental, consequential, indirect, or punitive damages as well as any circumstance for any complication, injuries, side effects or other medical accidents to person or property arising from or in connection with the use or reliance upon any information contained herein.

e) The author is not responsible for the contents of any linked site or any link contained in a linked site, or any changes or update to such sites. The inclusion of any link does not imply endorsement by the author. The author makes no representations or claims as to the quality, content and accuracy of the information, services, products, messages which may be provided by such resources, and specifically disclaims any warranties, including but not limited to implied or express warranties of merchantability or fitness for any particular usage, application or purpose.

f) The information provided is general in nature and is intended for educational and informational purposes only. It is not intended to replace or substitute the evaluation, judgment, diagnosis, and medical or preventative care of a physician, paediatrician, therapist and/or health care provider.

g) Any medical, nutritional, dietetic, therapeutic or other decisions, dosages, treatments or drug regimes should be made in consultation with a health care practitioner. Do not discontinue treatment or medication without first consulting your physician, clinician or therapist.

h) By reading this information, you signify your assent to these terms and conditions of use. If you do not agree to these terms and conditions of use, do not read/use this information. If any provision of these terms and conditions of use shall be determined to be unlawful, void or for any reason unenforceable, then that provision shall be deemed severable from this agreement and shall not affect the validity and enforceability of any remaining provisions.

i) The information, services, products, messages and other materials, individually and collectively, are provided with the understanding that the author is not engaged in rendering medical advice or recommendations.

j) The information and the terms of use are subject to change without notice. The material provided as is without warranty of any kind and may include inaccuracies and/or typographical errors. The author makes no representations about the suitability of this information for any purpose. The author disclaims all warranties with regard to this information, including all implied warranties, and in no event shall the author be held liable, resulting from, or in any way related to, the use of this information.

k) The unauthorized alteration of the content of this information is expressly prohibited. The author, its agents and representatives shall not be responsible for any claims, actions or damages which may arise on account of the unauthorized alteration of this information.

9 798215 730454